What You Eat Can Hurt You!

Learn Which Foods to Avoid and Which Ones to Eat to Stamp Out Inflammation, Illness and Disease, and to Stay Healthy!

RON KNESS

Cover Photo Credit - © Can Stock Photo Inc. / ifong

ISBN-13: 978-1500918880
ISBN-10: 1500918881

Disclaimer

This book has been written to provide information to help you learn how to fight disease by eating healthy. Every effort has been made to make this book as complete and accurate as possible. However, there may be mistakes in typography or content. Also, this book contains information on how to fight disease by eating healthy only up to the publishing date. Therefore, this book should be used as a guide – not as the ultimate source of learning how fight disease with healthy food.

The purpose of this book is to educate. The author and publisher do not warrant the information contained in this book is fully complete and shall not be responsible for any errors or omissions. The author and publisher shall have neither liability nor responsibility to any person or entity with respect to any loss or damage caused or alleged to be caused directly or indirectly by this book. If you do not wish to be bound by the above, please return this guide for a full refund.

Contents

A Message from the Author

FREE BONUS - The Healthy Lifestyle Report

Hey gang ... If you would like to learn even more about weight loss and living the healthy lifestyle, consider signing up for my free report.

It is 21 pages filled with tips and techniques you can use to further improve your weight loss and get healthy.

For a limited time, you can get this report delivered to your inbox by clicking on this link:
http://www.newplr4you.com/healthylifestyle/wp-content/uploads/2014/01/21st_Century_Nutrition_Ebook%20/Stick_to_Your_Healty_Lifestyle_Eating_Plan.pdf.

Health Mismanagement in Today's Society

We live in a society today where most healthcare practitioners would rather treat a symptom, condition, illness or disease instead of trying to prevent it in the first place. So as a healthcare consumer, you have to educate yourself so that

1) you can stay as healthy as possible so you don't need to have a doctor treat you and

2) if you do get sick, know all the your options available, including the natural ones which in many cases are just as effective.

Once you are sick is not the time to learn what you should have done that could have prevented it – take the preventative approach now to maintain your health into the future and if you do have any health issuing creeping up on you, to treat them now before they turn into something more serious later.

Preventative Medicine? Not Something Doctors Readily Discuss With You.

As we said, today's medicine is about treating instead of proactive prevention. How many times has your doctor discussed what you can do to stay healthy – especially when it comes to food and its preparation?

However, in their defense, they just do not have the time necessary with a waiting room full of ill patients to help. I know my doctor works on 15-minute appointments.

Unless you have something wrong with you, you most likely won't even get an appointment.

And from the pharmaceutical side of the house, there isn't any money in well patients. They make money when your doctor prescribed something to help or cure you after a health issue has taken hold. It is not in their best interest financially to keep you well!

So in the end, it is up to you to take control of your health. In this book we try to educate you on how you can stay well in the first place, but if you do get sick, foods you can eat to fight the disease, illness or condition. The Native Americans were (and many still are) very good at using foods to prevent and treat sickness, so it can be done. While we are going to go that deep into it, we are going to learn a little bit about using food to keep well and to get you well if you do get sick.

Know Your Options

Natural ways exist to treat various ailments. I would rather take my chance on holistic types of medicine instead of some of the pharmaceuticals that are out there. If you watch the advertisements, many times the side effects are worse than the condition it is treating!

Food is a natural source of both prevention and healing. Eating the right foods can help you develop an immunity to keep disease at bay before it has a chance to get hold in your body.

But there are also other alternative and holistic measures that a natural medicine doctor might prescribe. Depending on your illness, disease or condition, you might choose a blend of natural and traditional treatment.

For example, there really isn't an alternative to the traditional way of getting your kids vaccinated to help protect them from disease. But you can teach them the natural way of washing their hands to prevent the spread of germs. And, armed with the knowledge in this book, you can now feed them natural immune-boosting foods that help keep them healthy and protected against germ attacks.

Another example is trying to prevent cancer. You need to eat food high in anti-oxidants (the natural medicine way of prevention), along with getting periodic cancer screenings to catch any form of the disease that may have invaded your body (using traditional preventative medicine).

If you do develop cancer, you'll want to get the best traditional medical treatment available to you, but to increase your chances to survive, you'll also want to know what foods will help cure you and also the alternative and natural treatments that are proven to work.

Boost Your Health the Natural Way

To stay as well as possible, or to speed healing if you are sick, you need to do better manage these five things:

- Sleep

- Exercise

- Nutrition

- Stress

- Risky Behaviors

While we cover all five topics below, we spend more time on nutrition – the most important one of the five.

Sleep

Not getting enough sleep can lead to a whole host of medical issues ranging from chronic insomnia to increased risks of getting diabetes, high blood pressure and coronary disease. Studies have shown that sleep deprivation also causes high stress which itself can lead to depression. If left unchecked, depression can be a contributing cause of many health issues of its own including suicide.

To prevent a lack of sleep, first look at your surroundings. The temperature where you sleep should be slightly cool; it should also be quiet and dark.

You can control the temperature with fans and air conditioning, and darkness in the room with darkening window treatments, but you may not be able to do much about noise other than wearing ear plugs to bed. Also evaluate your mattress and pillows; are they supporting you correctly? If not, replace them. You should replace your mattress at least every eight years anyway.

Next look at your routine before you go to bed. What you do should unwind you and prepare you to sleep, not wind you up so you can't sleep. Some good ways to decompress include reading a book or taking a hot bath. Both do a good job at relaxing you. If you still are not sleeping enough at night, then maybe it is a nutrition issue that is preventing you from sleeping.

Try eating foods rich in antioxidants like vitamin C and selenium. These include green and red peppers, broccoli, cabbage and cauliflower for vegetables and strawberries, cantaloupe and oranges for fruits; seafood (tuna, halibut and shrimp) and meats like chicken and beef have selenium.

But what happens if you are getting enough sleep but still feel tired the next day? It could be a quantity verses quality issue. You are getting enough sleep hour-wise, but not enough good deep REM sleep.

To increase your sleep quality add some turkey and eggs to your last meal Eating an ounce of dark chocolate bar (at least 70% cocoa) also helps.

Exercise

We know exercise is a natural way to prevent disease and in many cases can reverse some health issues, such as heart disease and high blood pressure. But did you know it can also reverse diabetes? With a combined cardio/strength training program and healthy nutrition plan, many people no longer need to take insulin.

Exercise has also been found to reduce the risk of colon cancer and strengthen bones – the latter lowering the risk of osteoporosis.

Nutrition and exercise go hand-in-hand. Not only does the proper nutrition power you through your workouts, but it also helps your body recover afterward too.

An exercise/nutrition plan should include complex carbohydrates for the energy to get you through a workout and protein to help repair your muscles after a strength training session.

Nutrition

We cover this topic in much more detail later on in this book, but for now, let's say that in addition to repairing muscles and its other healing properties, nutrition can also strengthen your immune system, help your boost your memory and keep many of the major diseases at bay - heart disease, diabetes and cancer – all at the cellular level by just eating the right types of food.

Stress

Fact – 70 to 90% of all doctor's visits today originate issues caused by stress. In our busy world, stress is one of the primary issues that causes poor health in men, women, and sadly enough, even children.

Stress starts as a mental reaction to something that happens to you. As a result your mind tells your body to dump the hormone cortisol into your bloodstream. If you get this "fight or flight" hormone too often, it starts to take a toll on your body and you increase your risk for disease.

For example, stress:

- affects your insulin level

- can raise your blood pressure to dangerous levels

- increases your chance of a cancer taking hold

Stress is also linked to many of the common health issues too, such as:

- Flu

- Insomnia

- Digestive issues

- Urinary problems

- Infertility

- Headaches

Regardless, you have to get your stress under control before it degrades your health even more than what it already may have done. Fortunately, you have many natural options to help:

exercise to release endorphins – the "feel good" hormone and the anti-venom of cortisol,

mind relaxation techniques such as yoga,

aromatherapy, massage, and certain types of food.

Risky Behaviors

If you engage in any of the risky behaviors below, the best thing you can do for your health is to eliminate them:

- Drinking alcohol to excess
- Smoking
- Doing drugs
- Risky sex

Drinking Alcohol to excess

While drinking one or two drinks per day does have heart health benefits, drinking to excess frequently only increases your risk for disease.

Smoking

Smoking is never good – period. We now know it is not only harmful to you, but also to those around you that happen to inhale secondhand smoke. By smoking you could get lung disease or lung cancer, or heart disease.

Doing drugs

Prescription or illegal, this dangerous practice will eventually take a toll on your body. They weaken your body so your cells can't resist or recover from disease or infections.

Risky sex

Risky sexual behaviors are so very dangerous. With HIV rampant in some areas, not to mention all of the other STDs out there, always wear protection when with an unknown partner.

By eliminating risky behaviors from your lifestyle, you increase your chances of staying well and reversing disease if one does take hold. Once you are rid of these things, now is the time to start managing your health the natural way.

A good place to start is with what you eat (or don't eat). Nutrition is a powerful weapon against disease – and being it is something you do each day, why not eat things that are good for you and promote good health instead of junk that can hurt you or even lead to an early death?

The key is knowing which nutrients to add to your menu so that you can optimize your health. By giving your cells a chance to repair themselves and flushing toxins out of your body, you are giving yourself the best chance to succeed at good long-term health.

Fight Disease with Proper Nutrition

When you're ready to adopt a healthy lifestyle, you'll use food as fuel for your body, as a means to prevent disease and to heal yourself. On the nutrition side of your new lifestyle, you'll consciously know what food goes in your mouth, which foods not to eat and you will be constantly looking for natural ways to improve your health, such a limiting your intake of sugar, salt and the bad fats – saturated and trans.

Don't Eat Foods That Are Bad for Your Body

That seem like a simple enough statement doesn't it. However, in our world of processed food, what you may think is not bad for you may be loaded with things that if fact harmful to your body. If you don't start with raw ingredients and cook it yourself, you don't know for sure what is in it – especially if you eat in a restaurant. Even nutritional labels don't tell the whole story as evidenced by the paragraph below on trans-fat.

Trans Fat

If you buy processed foods, read the labels first. And don't make assumptions. For example if you see a nutrition label with 0 grams of trans-fat, add up the saturated and unsaturated grams and compare your total with the total fat listed.

If there is a difference of a ½ gram of less, the difference is most likely trans-fat – the worst kind. To find out if it is trans or not, go to the ingredients list and look for the words "hydrogenated" or "partially hydrogenated". If you see either, it is trans-fat. Here in the United States, the FDA allows food manufacturers to not list trans-fat if it is a half a gram of less.

And sometimes we just don't recognize a food that we were raised on as being bad. For example, take the lowly doughnut. They are good to eat, sweet and flavorful, but they are loaded with saturated fat, trans-fat and sugar.

Now I'm not saying you can never have a doughnut again, but I am saying to limit yourself to one now and then. As long as you account for it in your daily calories and saturated fat count, eating one once in a while is fine. My wife and I like to stop and get a doughnut at Wall Drug when going through Wall South Dakota. However, that is the only time we ever eat doughnuts, so we treat ourselves when making our yearly pilgrimage to Minnesota and back.

Monosodium Glutamate

Monosodium Glutamate or MSG is another culprit we should not eat. It was frequently found in certain types of Asian freshly prepared foods, although many restaurants have now stopped using it. You can also find it in processed meats, and canned products such as soups and vegetables.

Some people have a negative reaction to MSG in the form of headaches, nausea, fatigue, chest pain and more.

This is your body telling you it is a toxin and you should not be eating it. Even if you do not react to MSG, cut it out of your diet as much as possible.

Salt

We need a certain amount of salt in our body to maintain the proper electrolytes, however, many of us get way too much per day. The guidelines recommend no more than 2,300 milligrams per day, if under 50 years old and no more than 1,500 milligrams per day, if over 50.

Almost all that we eat, even sweet things, have a certain amount of salt in them, so we get more than enough already in the food we eat without adding more. Salt is a balancing game – you don't want too little, but yet you don't want too much either. Continually being at one extreme or the other and you can suffer negative health effects.

Sugar

Sugar is found in many foods – even those that seem healthy like the low-fat and light varieties. A food may tout that it has no added sugar, but if it is sweet, it is most likely sweetened with a sugar substitute which can be worse for you than real sugar. At least with real sugar, you know it is natural and what is in it. Here again is a case of learning how to read labels and understanding what they mean. About the only safe sugar substitute is from the stevia plant. Truvia® is one commonly available product derived from this plant.

Americans typically eat up to 3 pounds of sugar per person *per week*. According to the American Heart Association, men should eat about 37.5 grams (or about 9 teaspoons or 150 calories) per day; women, 25 grams per day (6 teaspoons or 100 calories per day). At 3 pounds per week, that is 181 grams per day or almost 5 times the daily recommended amount for a man and 4 ½ times for a women.

Sugar is not only making us fat, but unhealthy. It damages your immune system, boosts your risk of heart disease and eventually leads to Type 2 diabetes.

Gluten

Gluten can be a problem for some people. Found in many grains, including whole ones, they should be an important ingredient in your healthy eating plan, if you are not gluten-reactive. If you are, then you are better off eating gluten-free grains, such as corn, quinoa, wild rice, millet, and buckwheat.

Learn to Eat Healthy the Mediterranean Way

By far, the best diet you can follow is the healthy Mediterranean-style. It is by far the heart healthiest of all eating plans, because it gives your body what it needs to maintain good overall health.

Heart-healthy, the diet consists of:

- Fruits

- Vegetables

- Whole Grains

- Nuts

- Olive Oil

- Seeds

- Legumes

- Beans

- Herbs and Spices

In addition to this basic diet, you should supplement it with:

- healthy fish high in Omega 3 a couple of times a week, such as tuna, herring, halibut or mackerel;

- low-fat dairy;

- poultry periodically, such as the white meat of chicken or turkey;

- and lean red meat.

If disease has already hit your life, then you have to eat differently. Let's look at five common health issues and see how eating healthy can treat the disease or even cure you:

- Diabetes

- Heart Disease

- Inflammation

- Alzheimer's Disease

- Cancer

Diabetic Nutritional Management

Managing and treating diabetes is not about cutting sugar out of your diet forever, but maintaining a stable blood sugar level. In certain people with hypoglycemia, they actually have to eat sugar to get their glucose level up to a safe level. This condition can be caused by overmedicating with too much insulin.

It can be just as dangerous as hyperglycemia – too high of a glucose level. Both conditions can be life-threatening if left untreated.

So not only is managing diabetes about what you eat, but also when you eat. The goal is to keep a stable glucose level. Blood sugar levels should be maintained between 70-130 mg/dL on a regular basis. A spike should not go above 180 mg/dL a couple of hours after you eat.

By eating in moderation and losing weight, diabetes can actually reverse itself so the person is no longer dependent on insulin.

What Not to Eat

As a diabetic, you have to learn to make better food choices. When possible, select diabetic-friendly options that are low on the Glycemic Index so your blood sugar doesn't spike.

Below is a partial list of foods you **do not** want to eat as they raise your blood sugar level too high:

- White bread

- Pasta

- White potatoes

- Popcorn

- Candy

- Cereal

- Watermelon

- Pineapple

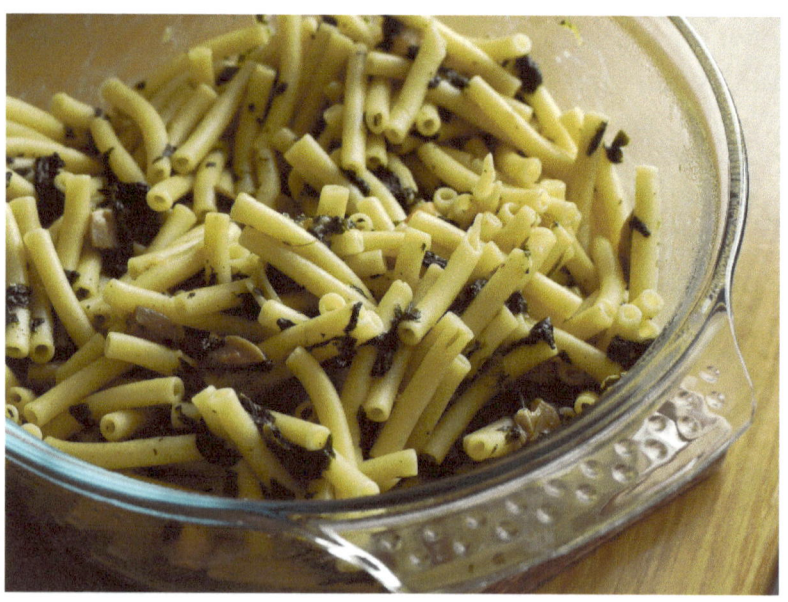

If you happen to eat a food high on the scale, balance it off with a food listed lower. Also, watch your portions of high glycemic index foods – eat only a little bit.

If your favorite foods happen to be high on the list, don't forbade them forever – just each a small portion now and then to keep your cravings at bay.

As far as beverages, your best bet is to drink water – plenty of water. Sugary drinks are out as you can imagine, and so are fruit juices. While they may sound healthy, they are loaded with sugar – even if it is a natural type of sugar, it can still cause problems for a diabetic.

Eat These Foods to Keep Your Diabetes In Check

Now that you know what not to eat, how about what you can eat. Dark, leafy green vegetables are a great addition to your meal plan. For a real breakfast treat, add spinach to your omelet or scrambled eggs or eat a side salad with your main entree. Spinach is a super food that keeps you full longer, is carb friendly and low in calories.

Kale is another leafy green to eat. Also try mustard greens, collard greens, and turnip greens to see if any of these appeal to your palate.

Tomatoes are a healthy option for diabetics because they're full of vitamins and nutrients, such as vitamin E and C and iron. You can eat them sliced raw, in soup or as a tomato sauce over whole wheat pasta. If you buy tomato sauce, be sure to check how much sugar is in it. If you make your own, you can leave the sugar out.

Beans are a great food for everybody, but especially diabetics. They are packed with protein, fiber, potassium and magnesium and they keep you full longer than many other vegetables. Because you can get your protein from beans, you won't have to eat as much meat, meaning you'll eat less saturated fat.

Regular potatoes generally are not a good choice for diabetics, however sweet potatoes are another superfood you can eat. Sweet potatoes good for a diabetic that shouldn't to have much for sweets. Who would have guessed!

Sweet potatoes are low on the GI scale, but packed with fiber, vitamin A and many other nutrients good for you. You can microwave a whole sweet potato or cut them up into fries and bake them in the oven.

To make great fries, cut them into ¼" strips. Put them on a rack that fits inside of a cookie sheet and spray with a non-stick cooking spray. Mix up a seasoning for them by combining salt, thyme or rosemary, course ground black pepper, sweet paprika and cayenne pepper to taste. Bake at 450° until done. They are a very healthy alternative to French fries.

When it comes to fruit, not all fruit is good for a diabetic person to eat. But some can help – such as citrus options – oranges, grapefruit, and even lemons and limes – which you can put in your water for a flavorful option. You get fiber and vitamin C – and it helps boost your immune system in the process.

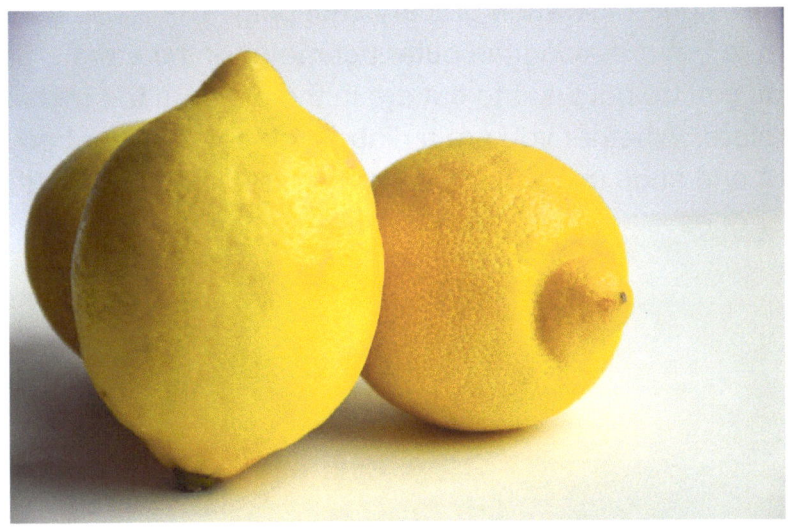

As far as bread, a better option for diabetics is one made out of whole grain. Be sure to read the nutrition label so you know how much sugar is in it. With whole grains, you'll get some omega-3 fatty acids, folate and chromium that your body can use to help heal itself.

Other foods that are diabetic-friendly are:

- berries (all kinds)

- walnuts

- flax seeds

You can have some dairy products, but make sure they don't have added sugar. You need the vitamin D for strong bones and healthy teeth that dairy provides, but yet you don't want a blood sugar spike. A very good alternative that we drink all the time is unsweetened almond milk. Not on is it good tasting, at only 30 calories per serving, it is waist-friendly too.

I'll share one trick when grocery shopping. The foods you need to eat are along the outer perimeter of the store. The foods you do not want to eat are in the aisles in the middle of the store. Whether you are a diabetic or not, do your body a favor and shop more along the outer aisles and less on the inner ones.

Prevent and Reverse Heart Disease the Natural Way

Heart disease sneaks up on you. You generally don't know you have it until you start experiencing symptoms. Whether you already have it, and are trying to manage it, or you don't have it and want to prevent getting it, food can play a big part in each instance.

The number one killer of both men and women in the United States, heart disease happens when your arteries become partially to fully blocked by accumulated plaque. If you are not showing signs of the disease yet, then you definitely want to follow a diet that:

1) keeps plaque from forming and

2) breaks up what has already formed so it doesn't cause trouble down the road.

Prevent Plaque by Eliminating These Foods from Your Diet

The first thing you want to manage, in terms of food, is portion size. Your body can handle a little bit of unhealthy food once in a while. It can become overwhelmed when you eat super-sized portions of food not good for you too often.

If you're used to eating large portions, it is tough to just cut back cold turkey. Instead, eliminate the unhealthy food and replace it with low calorie healthy foods like dark, leafy greens or cruciferous vegetables like cauliflower, cabbage or broccoli. You can basically have an unlimited amount of these so you can still get filled up, but without all the things that are not good for you.

We talked about cutting out the things that are bad for you to eat. The first two things that come to mind are trans-fat and saturated fat. These two fats are found in things such as processed foods (think hot dogs, deli meats and sandwich meats) and fried foods (doughnuts, French fries, State Fair foods).

Of the two, you should avoid trans-fat as much as you can. Because it is a manufactured fat, the body does not know how to break it down, so it stores it as fat. Read the label; if it has "hydrogenated" or "partially hydrogenated" anywhere in the ingredients, it has trans-fat in it.

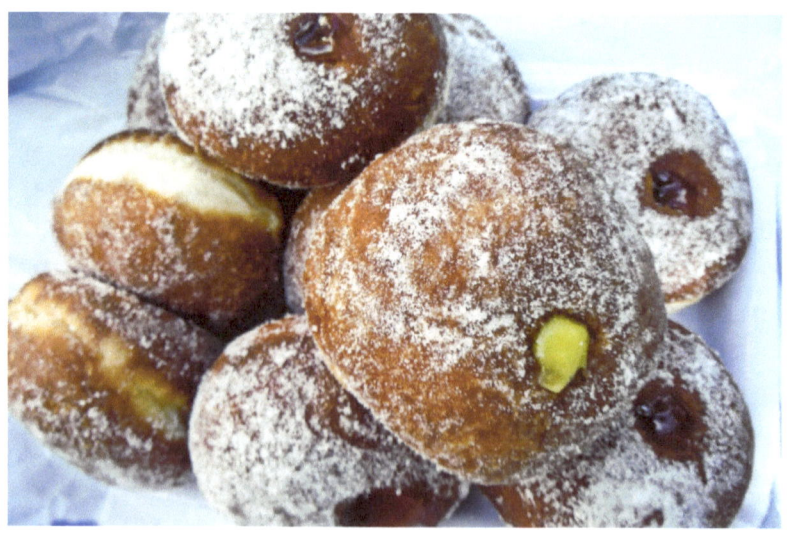

Marbled red meat and whole dairy products, including ice cream and cheese, also have a lot of saturated fat. Fortunately both have better healthier options – lean red meat along with chicken and turkey, and lots of skim, fat-free, 1% or 2% dairy options.

When cooking meals, you want to avoid using fats that are solid at room temperature, like butter and margarine, and instead use healthier alternatives such as olive oil, canola or safflower/sunflower oils. I cover the topic of healthy cooking more in the last chapter of this book.

When buying food at the grocery store, buy fresh ingredients when possible. Prepackaged foods are normally high in sodium which is bad for your heart. Learn to read nutrition labels and know what the information means.

Avoid buying pre-packed vegetables that are drowning in cream-based sauces or fruit canned with added sugar or high fructose syrup. If you can't get fresh, then choose frozen vegetables – just plain vegetables without any added sauce. In fruits, choose ones that are packed in their own juices.

Grains are an essential staple in any heart-healthy diet plan, but be sure yours are whole grain. Processed grains, like the enriched white flour found in white breads, cakes and biscuits have been stripped of the part that is good for you – the fiber and other essential nutrients.

Your goal for your healthy diet should be eating foods that keep your bad LDL cholesterol low and your good HDL (good) cholesterol levels high.

Foods to **stay away from** include things we commonly eat such as:

- Cheese

- Pizza

- Desserts

- Marbled beef

- Whole milk

- White Pasta

- Candy

- Butter

When reading the above list, some healthy substitutes should come into mind, like using low fat cheese, lean meats, skim or 1% dairy and whole wheat pasta. See how easy it is to substitute healthy options for foods that are bad for you!

Boost Your Heart Health with These Foods

Some foods can start out perfectly fine, but then are ruined due to the way they are prepared. For example taking the skin off of a chicken and either grilling or smoking it would be healthy, but leaving the skin on and frying it in shortening would not.

Another practice that lowers the fat content in food is if you make a soup or stew. Before reheating it, skim off the solidified fat and throw it away before reheating.

The best heart-healthy diet includes a balance if lean meats, fruits, vegetables, whole grains, nuts and seeds. As far as good grains to eat, look for:

- Whole grain bread and pasta

- High fiber cereal and oatmeal

- Brown rice

- Flaxseed

One of the main ingredients in your heart-healthy diet plan should be vegetables – especially those high in Vitamin B6 like asparagus and bell peppers. These two vegetables keep your homocysteine level low – something that contributes to heart disease. An easy way to choose vegetables is to look for a rainbow of color, such as:

- Orange – carrots

- Red – radishes and tomatoes

- Yellow – peppers, cauliflower

- Green – green beans, peppers, broccoli, celery, cabbage and others too numerous to name. Your goal should be to eat at least 8 servings of fresh fruits and vegetables per day - not canned or frozen options, unless nothing else is available.

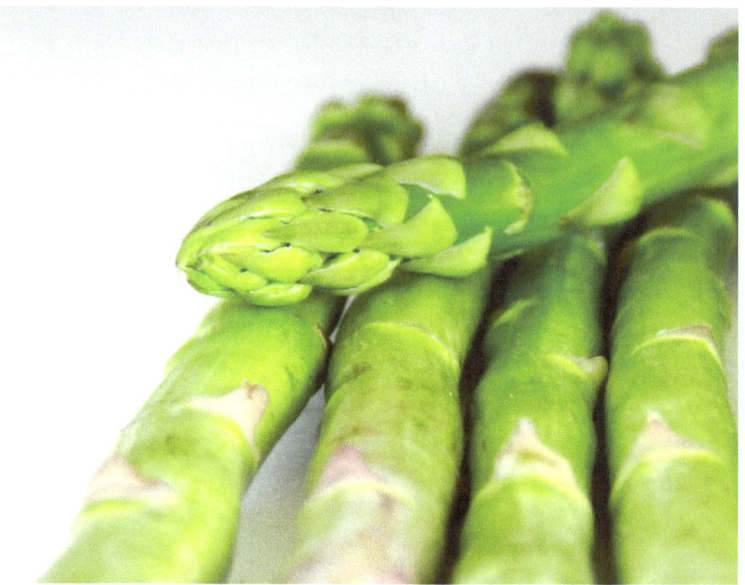

Tree nuts like almonds, pecans and walnuts – as well as seeds – are all good for your heart. They are filling, yet good for you as they are high in Omega 3. A handful of almonds for dessert would be a much better option than a slice of cake. Make sure to select raw nuts. When roasted, it can add saturated fat and usually salt.

Speaking of Omega-3, salmon and tuna are good choices for fish. For meats, look to the white meat of chicken and turkey, pork and lean cuts of beef. If you get ground beef, get at least 93% lean.

Managing your heart health is not hard once you realize what you should not be eating and instead what you should eat. Just a few simple tweaks here and there will make your current eating plan heart-healthy. Now add in some daily exercise and you are well on your way to reversing heart disease if you already have it or protecting yourself from getting it.

Take a Bite Out of Inflammation With Food

Granted inflammation isn't something that will kill you, but it can make you miserable and lessen your quality of life if you are in constant pain from it. I've been down that road with an inflamed bursa sac in both shoulders (fortunately not both at the same time). The last one took me two years to get rid of with physical therapy three times per week and proper eating.

Inflammation is your body's way of telling you something is wrong and that it is working to protect you – hence the pain. It is usually localized to just one area and is a response to something that is attacking you like bacteria or a virus.

But in its effort, inflammation usually results in pain, swelling and redness. The pain and swelling usually force you to go easy on that part of the body so it has time to heal.

Food to the rescue! Eating the right types of food can help alleviate the pain and swelling. By not eating certain foods that cause inflammation and eating foods that keep the inflammation at bay, you can get well quicker and get your quality of life back.

Foods That Cause Inflammation Flare-Ups

Below is a list of foods that can increase your chances of getting an inflammation. In keeping with our eliminate-and-replace regimen, you should avoid these foods as much as you can:

- Alcohol

- Fried foods

- Processed meats (bacon, hot dogs, bologna)

- Fried Eggs

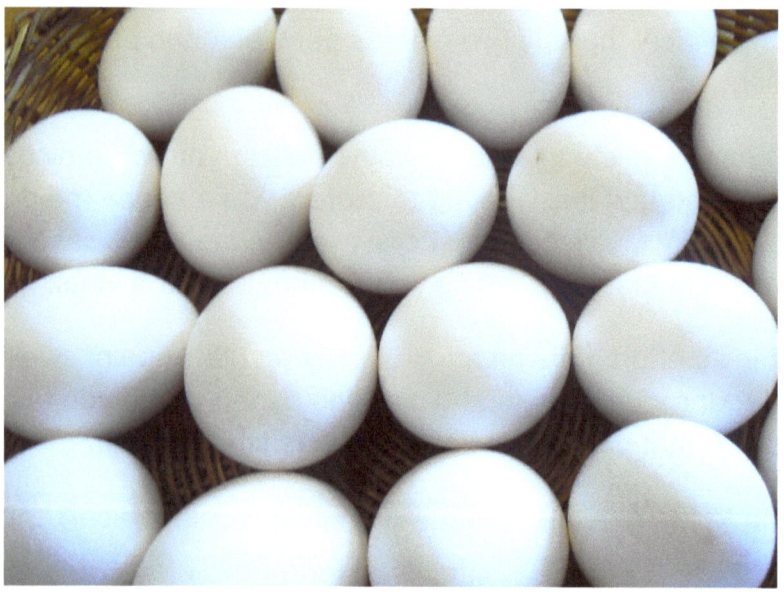

If you have arthritis, then you especially want to steer clear of foods on this list. A better choice overall would be to stick to the Mediterranean style diet which limits meat and focuses heavily on fruits, whole grains and vegetables instead.

Eat fresh when you can. Prepared foods high in salt, sugar and saturated fat can actually cause more pain in your body.

Minimize meat. Make it a small portion of your meal instead of the main entrée. The main culprit in meat is the arachidonic acid it contains; it can cause inflammation or worsen it if you already have it. Studies have shown that people who eat vegetarian and those who eat very little meat have a lower incidence of inflammation.

Full-fat dairy products can be hard on your body also. Choose low-fat, skim or the lower percent fat options in cheese, yogurt and milks.

Of course if you react to gluten found in wheat and many other products, you will want to eliminate these products from your diet to lessen the chance of a gluten reaction. There are lots of gluten-free products on the market with more showing up every day, so it is not hard to go gluten-free.

Eat These Non-Inflammatory Foods to Heal Your Body

The key to keeping inflammation at bay or even inflammation-free is to keep the body from attacking itself in the first place. This has to be done at the cellular level by eating foods from this list:

- Omega 3 - Choose any of the Omega-3 "fatty" fishes two to three times per week instead of marbled meats. These include salmon, tuna, mackerel and herring.

- Soy – Used as a meat substitute, soy helps lower inflammation in your body. Natural choices include tofu and edamame.

- Dark green leafy vegetables – You can't go wrong eating spinach, kale, turnip greens, collard greens or mustard greens. They have a positive effect on keeping inflammation down due to the large amount of Vitamin E.

- Low-fat dairy – A common misconception today is that all dairy is bad for you. Not true! You need dairy – just not the full-fat versions. Instead choose the low-fat options. Yogurt is a good choice because of the probiotics it contains. This helps keep down the bad bacteria in your intestinal track.

- Grains – Eat whole grain products. The fiber they contain helps suppress C-reactive protein, which can lead to inflammation flare-ups. If you already have an inflammation, whole grain can help reduce the pain and swelling.

- Nuts - Nuts are a great food because of the fiber, calcium, omega-3 fatty acids and vitamin E in them. The tree nuts – walnuts, almonds and pecans – are the best choices. The antioxidants in nuts help repair inflammation in your body.

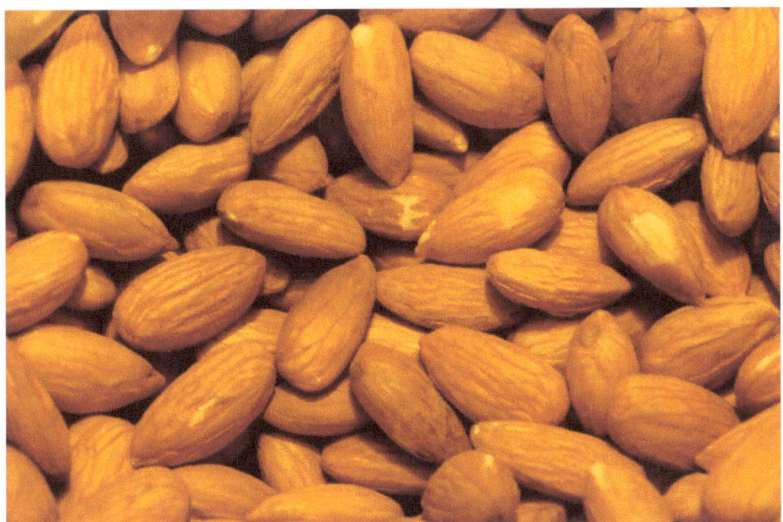

- Peppers – Who would have thought that peppers can actually help keep inflammation down! A good choice that aren't all that hot are bell peppers. They come in a variety of colors which can spruce up the appearance when used in a meal. Some spicy choices include peppers like chili, serrano, habanero or cayenne.

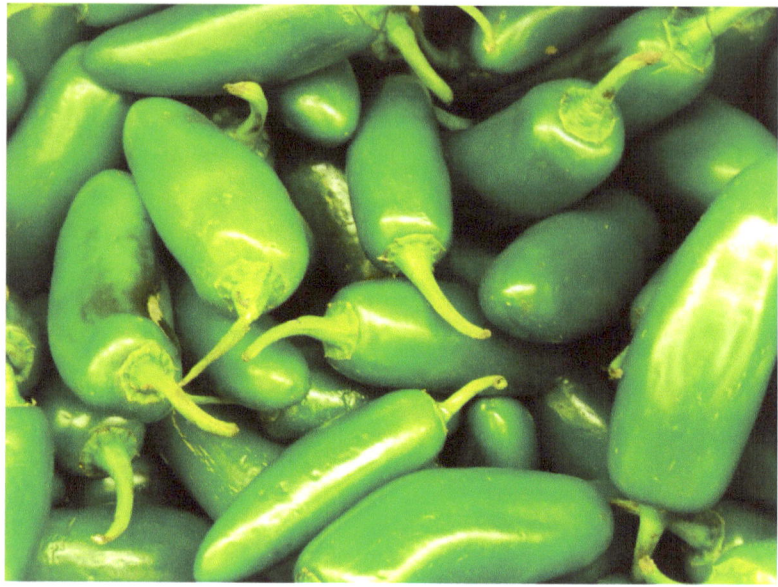

It is the capsaicin in peppers that help reduce pain and inflammation. It is so good that many of the topical creams and applications for arthritis include it.

While all of this is good information to know and try, you have to keep track of what works for you. Managing inflammation is not a one-size-fits-all solution. What works for you may not work for someone else.

In the end, either don't eat or at least eat less of foods that worsen or don't help your inflammation and eat more of what helps.

Remember, Nutrition Boosts Your Memory

Two of the most feared health issues today for many men and women is dementia and Alzheimer's disease. Because the loss of memory takes your identity with it, it is important to do everything you can to preserve your memories and to maximize brain function.

Many older people try to stay as sharp as they can by playing strategy games and puzzles that are supposed to help maintain mental clarity. But your choice of food can either help or hurt your memory retention attempts.

Flush Memory-Stealing Toxins Out of Your Body

The brain is very sensitive, so one thing that can cause irreparable damage is a lack of blood. This is usually associated with a build-up of plaque – the same thing that causes the narrowing of arteries as we discussed in the chapter on heart disease. So not only do you want to avoid those foods, but you want to eat food that can help boost your memory.

Eat These Foods to Increase Your Brain Function

If you are having trouble recalling your short or long-term memory, a B12 or iron deficiency could be the blame. Foods high in these two nutrients can help significantly. Seafood, fortified soy products, beef, lamb, dairy products and eggs all are rich in B12. Seafood, nuts, seeds, beef, lamb, beans, whole grains, tofu, dark leafy greens and cocoa powder are iron rich.

Did you see that seafood, beef and lamb are on both lists?

Antioxidants help preserve the connections of nerve cells in your brain. Foods high in antioxidants include: potatoes, pecans, cinnamon, red and black beans and all of the berries.

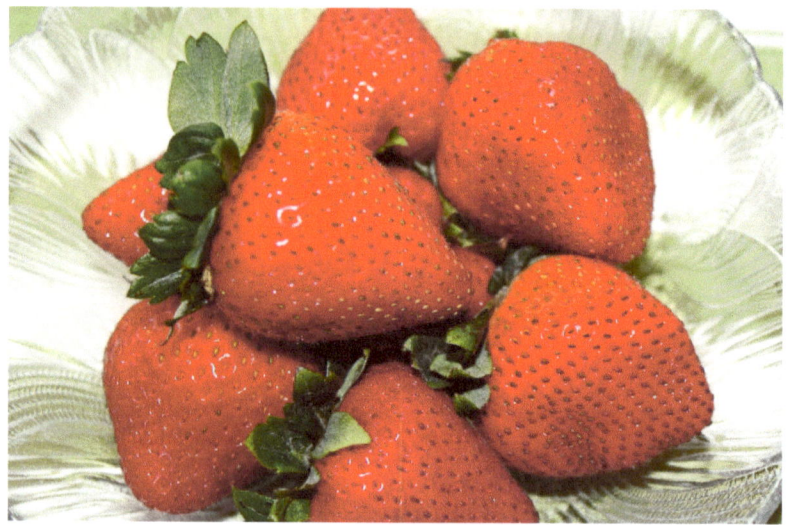

When you're starting to plan out your meals for the week, be sure to include foods from the above list that are high in B12, iron and antioxidants. They not only help keep brain cells healthy, but also maintain the vital nerve connections between the cells.

Anything you can do to help the flow of blood will generally help your brain, however flavonoids can also help boost your memory. Foods such as:

• Berries

• Apricots

• Pears

- Pinto and Black Beans

- Red Onions

- Apples

- Cabbage

- Tomatoes

- Parsley

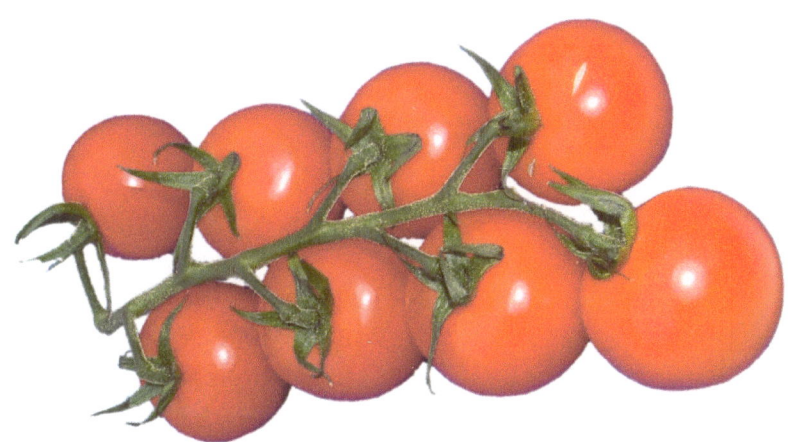

Folate has been found to help with brain function also. Foods high in folic acid with vitamin B12 includes:

- Spinach

- Asparagus

- White Navy Beans

- Lentils

- Broccoli

- Cereal fortified with folic acid

Finally sugar can potentially harm your memory. We are not talking about naturally occurring sugar like fresh fruit, but instead of the sugar in baked goods and soft drinks. Another memory stealer is trans-fat. This includes processed foods which are not only harmful nutritionally, but are harmful in repairing or retaining memory function.

And if you already have some memory damage, don't give up. It is never too late to start eating foods that can help retain what memory you have left or even help reverse a memory loss trend. And besides, it is just all good food to eat that is also good for you!

News Flash - Control and Cure Cancer Through Nutrition

Cancer. Without a doubt, it is the most feared word when it comes to medical issues. And cancer is non-discriminatory – it strikes both genders throughout the age groups. Regardless of the type of cancer or how early it is detected, the word drives a big stake right through our heart.

I think part of the fear comes from not knowing how to fully prevent it. If your risk is hereditary, there isn't much you can do to prevent it except get screened regularly. Early detection provides the best chance at curing it and can be life-saving in many instances. We also know that keeping fit and heart-healthy can help reduce your risk of cancer.

But what about food? How does that affect staying cancer free or helping recover from cancer? Not only does the food you eat or not eat have an effect on cancer, but studies show so does how it is prepared.

Grilling can increase your risk of cancer if you grill your meats until they are charred. Cooking meat at a high heat seems to be the culprit that can release or create cancer-causing chemicals. So if you grill, do so at a lower temperature and don't cook the meat until it is charred on the outside.

Get Rid of Cancer Causing Toxins

Processed meats, like sandwich meat, hot dogs, sausage and bacon can cause cancer. Not only are these meats filled with preservatives and additives, but many contain high levels of nitrates – especially bacon.

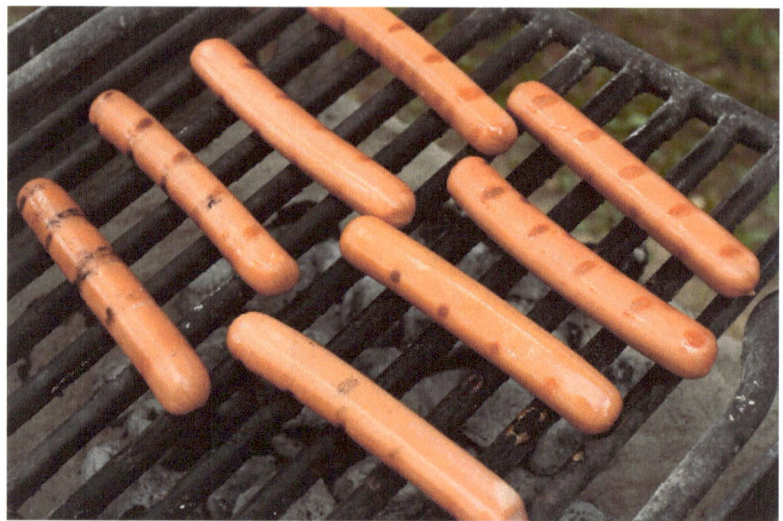

Studies have shown that people who eat a lot of processed meats are twice as likely to develop colorectal cancer and have increased risk of developing either stomach or pancreatic cancer. The culprit seems to be the nitrates. When ingested, they become nitrosamines.

And it just isn't processed meats. Red meat consumption has been linked to cancer too - prostate, colon and breast.

Fried foods can help contribute to cancer. So that doughnut you enjoy with your morning coffee probably isn't good for you, but then neither are the French fries or potato chips you eat at lunch either.

Finally, the last food we want to talk about is sugar. Not only does it contribute to obesity, but it also can contribute to the formation of cancer. If you already have cancer, sugar feeds the cells and makes them stronger, thus thwarting your efforts to eradicate them.

Studies prove that sugar and cancer have a connection. Both genders that consume foods high in sugar or high on the Glycemic Index have a higher risk of developing cancer, especially:

- Pancreatic

- Skin

- Uterine

- Urinary

- Breast

Cancer is the number 2 killer in the United States – heart disease is number 1. Don't give cancer what it needs to survive or develop. Now granted, the foods mentioned above in moderation aren't most likely not going to hurt you, but don't make a steady diet of consuming large quantities of them as you will be spinning the roulette wheel and like everything thing else in gambling, your luck will eventually run out.

Foods That Prevent the Growth of Cancer Cells

One of the best types of foods you can eat to protect yourself from the development or growth of cancer cells, are those high in antioxidants. They prevent or slow down oxidation that happens at the cellular level. It is the result of this oxidation process that gives cancer cells what they need to thrive inside your body, thus killing off healthy cells until you start developing symptoms of cancer. Stop the oxidation and you can stop the development of cancer.

Berries are strong antioxidants – with blueberries being the best and cranberries come a close second. Also grapefruit and oranges provide antioxidant protection. Besides antioxidants, it seems that Vitamin C plays a major role in keeping cancer cells at bay.

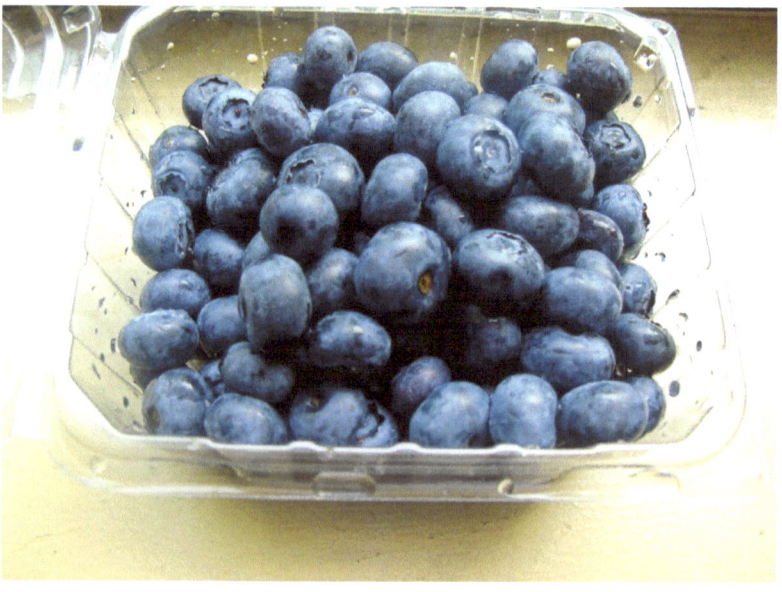

Certain vegetables are also known for their cancer fighting properties – especially bell peppers, broccoli and sweet potatoes.

And then there are herbs and spices. Not only do they make your food taste good, but they have anti-inflammatory agents and antioxidants, too.

Knowing what to eat and what to avoid seems to be one of the secrets to being cancer-free. As the saying goes "Knowledge is power." It is no truer than in health and the prevention of illness and disease.

Hopefully you have picked up on the trend in food in this book. Most of your diet should consists of:

- Fresh fruits, especially those high in Vitamin C and all of the berries

- Fresh vegetables, especially the dark leafy green and cruciferous ones

- Whole grains

- Raw nuts and seeds

- Lean meats

- Fatty fish

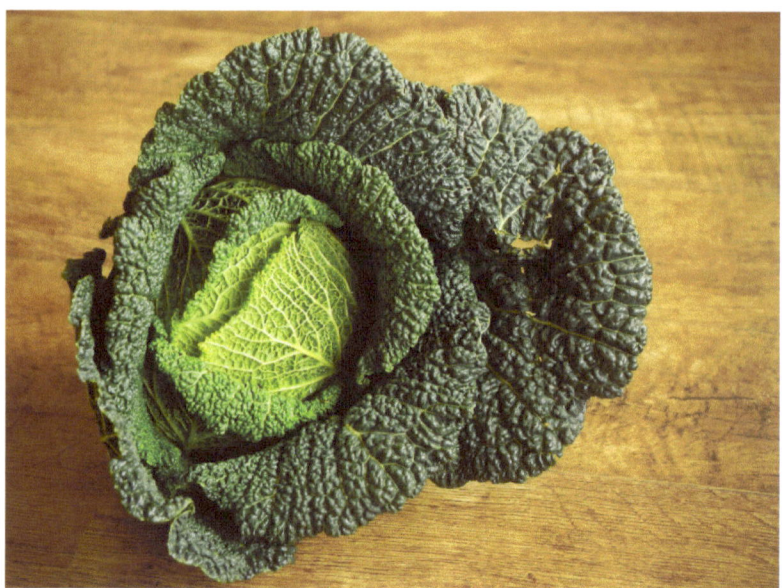

 If you concentrate your diet on this list, along with regular exercise, portion control and preparing your food as discussed in the next chapter, you will be doing as much as you can to stay healthy and free from illness and disease.

How to Cook Healthy

In the previous chapters, we looked at foods you should eat to stay healthy and foods you should avoid. But unless you eat only raw food, which is great for fresh fruits and vegetables but not so much for meats, you also have to know how to cook food properly. You might start with perfectly healthy food, but cook it wrong and it can do you more harm than good.

Below are six easy ways to prepare food to keep it healthy for you to eat. We start out with various cooking methods and then move on to cooking meats, which fats to cook with, cooking whole grains and vegetables and wrap it up by little tweaks you can make to your recipes to make them healthy. So let's get started.

Cooking Methods

There are many ways you can cook something. You might microwave it, or steam, bake, grill or use a variety of other cooking methods. The method you use can greatly increase or decrease the healthiness of the final product.

Microwaving

A general misconception is that microwaving food is bad for you. Wrong! The method of cooking isn't bad – it is usually the food microwaved that is bad even before it is cooked. Think about it, what do most people cook in a microwave?

Quick and easy (and processed) meals they take out of the freezer and in a few minutes have something to eat.

We know most of those meals are packed with refined grains, less than desirable cuts of fatty meat and generally loaded with sugar, saturated fat and trans-fat.

But what if you lightly cooked raw vegetables in your microwave? A few minutes in the microwave can soften up your vegetables without cooking out all of the nutrients as other cooking methods can do such a boiling. Now you have a new piece of equipment that you can use to cook healthy.

Steaming

When lightly steamed, vegetables retain their nutrients, as they don't set in water while cooking. Generally speaking vegetables should be cooked until you can just easily run a fork through them. Of course you can overcook vegetables in a steamer, so you have to watch how long you cook them. A good steamer is cheap to buy and most of them have a good manual with times to cook different things. Use that information as a starting point and adjust your times to the amount of doneness you want.

Vegetables cooked in a steamer can be bland, but it is easy to perk up the flavor by adding a little healthy olive oil. Also don't overlook adding in some seasonings or spices. Seasonings such as the ones made by Dash add a lot of flavor, but without the salt.

Baking

This is another tried-and-true healthy method of cooking. The key to baking is to not overcook. Cook until just done and then take it out. Baking helps keep in the flavor and natural juices, but you'll lose some of the nutrients due to the long baking time of most foods.

Grilling

A summertime method of cooking, not only is grilling a great way to cook meats and vegetables, but it can become a social gathering point around the grill. Grilling tends to cook out the fat in meat while at the same time locking in the taste.

Most food is grilled on grates which allow the fat to drip down and away from food. This makes your food even healthier by eradicating the saturated fat out of it. Just be sure not to char it.

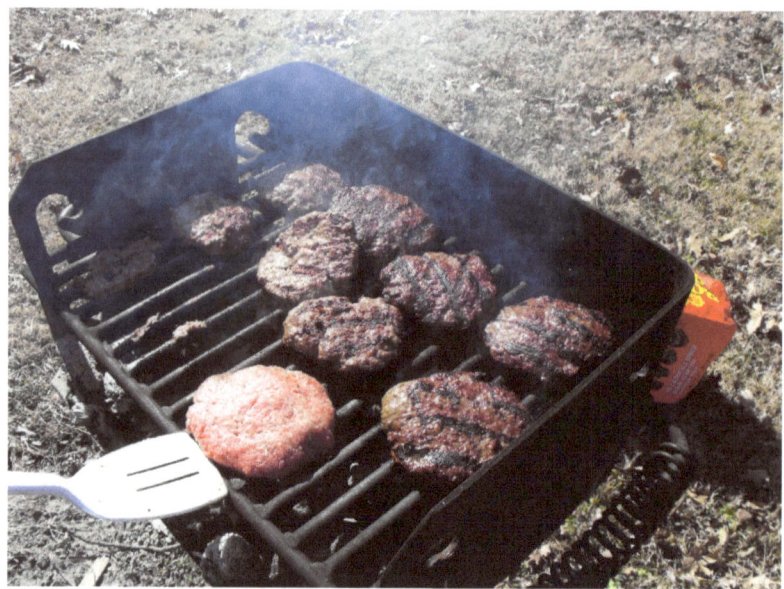

Boiling and frying

These two methods are generally the least preferable, because they either decrease the nutrients in your food (as with boiling) or add fat to your food (as with frying). However, there are ways to use these methods and still cook healthy.

Take frying for example. You can do it healthy or unhealthy depending on what you use to fry your food in. If you use a solid fat such as lard, bacon grease or shortening, then your food will be unhealthy. However if you use an oil that is liquid at room temperature , such as olive oil, canola oil or a sunflower or safflower oil, then you can make it healthy. Just know that frying is the least desirable of all the cooking methods.

Now, let's look at some ways to cook specific types of foods.

Meat

While some people are ok with being vegetarians or vegan, many people like to have meat with their meals. If you are a "meat" person, then learning how to cook it healthy is important.

Start with an organic meat if available. This ensures the animal was not fed hormones or feed that was unhealthy for them. Animals that were free-range or fed organic feed will be healthier for you to consume.

Granted, organic meat does cost more, but what price can you pay for health? If you end up getting ill or a disease from unhealthy eating, your medical bills will far outweigh the little bit of extra cost for organic meat.

Once you find a good selection of organic meat, make your selection better by the cut of meat you choose. Lean cuts with little to no marbling are the best for you.

The trick to cooking lean cuts of meat is to select good meat to begin with. Let's look at some ways to do this:

- **Hamburger** – Most meat counters offer a selection of different lean to fat ratios. While you may have bought 80/20 in the past, you should look at buying hamburger with the least amount of fat, such as 93/7 or 95/5.

- **Chicken and Turkey**– Generally you want to buy skinless cuts or cut off the skin after you get home prior to cooking it. White meat is generally healthier than dark meat.

- **Fish** – The "fatty four" saltwater fishes are the best to eat due to the high amount of Omega-3 they contain. Choose tuna, herring, halibut or mackerel.

Fats

As discussed earlier in this book, some fats are actually good for you – the unsaturated mono and polys. You need fats to stay healthy. Some vitamins are fat-soluble so without fat, those would be flushed out of your system. The trick is knowing which ones to cook with and which ones are best avoided.

A good rule of thumb is if a fat is solid at room temperature, it is one that you do not want to use. Liquid olive oil is much healthier than a stick of butter. Other good choices are canola oil, sunflower oil and safflower. Coconut oil and palm oils sound like they would be healthy, but they should be avoided as they contain a lot of saturated fat.

Grains

When it comes to grains, the only ones that are healthy are those in their natural state – unrefined and non-processed. Look for breads that contain whole grain. Many of them now how the whole grain stamp on the outside of the package and the number of grams of whole protein each serving has in it.

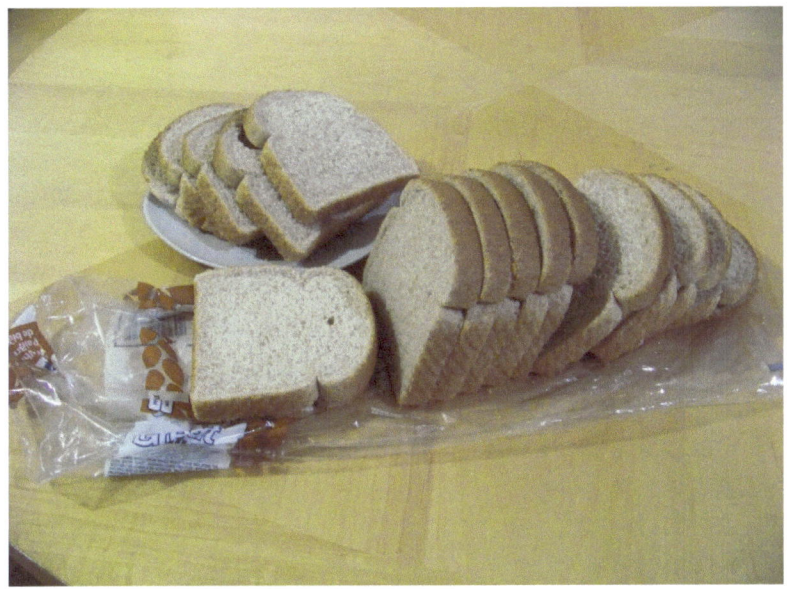

There are many choices of whole grains to choose from besides whole wheat and oats. One fairly new one on the market that you may not have tried yet is quinoa. It is great as a side dish or when used as part of a recipe requiring whole grain. Other great grains include:

- Bulgar

- Brown Rice

- Barley

- Rye

- Buckwheat

- Couscous

- Freekeh

- Spelt

Vegetables

Steamed or sautéed are two good ways to cook vegetables as far as retaining flavor and nutrients. The less you cook vegetables, the better they are for you.

Unlike many other foods, vegetables are great when eaten raw. Try that with a piece of steak! There are so many good vegetables that are best when eaten raw including:

- baby spinach

- turnips

- cauliflower

- broccoli

- carrots

- and so many more too numerous to name.

And vegetables are loaded with antioxidants which are good to keep down inflammation and the formation of cancer cells.

Recipe Tweaks for Improved Health

You most likely have some great recipes that have been handed down through the generations. However, many of those recipes are high in salt, sugar, or saturated fat. People were not conscious of those three unhealthy items back in their time. However, with a little work, you can make healthy versions of these recipes without sacrificing flavor.

For example, if a recipe calls for one egg, use two egg whites instead. If you want to retain the yellow color, add just half a yolk. Recipes calling for sour cream or cottage cheese are easy to "healthify". There are low-fat or reduced fat versions of both. Avoid using fat-free as that can change the outcome of the recipe.

Instead of using prepackaged seasonings that are usually loaded with salt, try adding in your own fresh seasonings. We have stopped using packaged chili and taco seasonings opting instead to make our own. After some trial-and-error, we have come up with both great tasting recipes that are equally good, if not better, than the prepackaged mixes.

Conclusion

Now you know what kinds of food you should eat - and what not to eat - as far as staying healthy or battling an inflammation, illness, disease or condition. Use common sense though. If you suspect you have something major, by all means go to a doctor. You may need to fight it both the traditional way using treatments and medicines along with the natural way with food.

However, the foods discussed in this book are part of a healthy-lifestyle plan for "clean" eating. So even if you have nothing wrong with you, these foods will keep you healthy and when eaten in conjunction with an exercise program, allow you to lose weight.

If you did not pick up on it, there was a common thread woven throughout the book – most of your food should be:

- Fresh fruits and vegetables,

- Lean meats,

- The big four fatty fishes,

- Nut and seeds,

- Whole grains,

- Reduced fat dairy,

- Healthy oils high in mono and poly unsaturated fats.

If most of your food comes from this list, you should stay healthy for a long time and enjoy a great quality of life.

Other Healthy Books By the Author

Hi, I'm Ron. If you enjoyed this book, I invite you to look at my other healthy eating/healthy lifestyle selections. Depending on if you have a lot of weight to lose, a little to lose or you just want to know how to cook and eat healthier, I have a book that covers the topic.

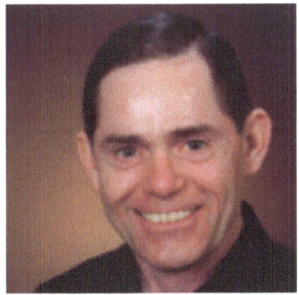

Now onto my other books!

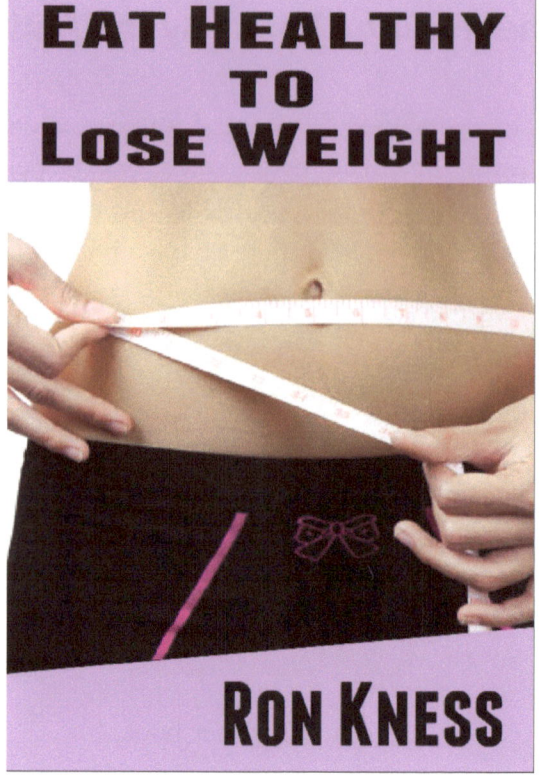

Eat Healthy to Lose Weight
at
http://www.amazon.com/Eat-Healthy-Lose-Weight-Traditional-
ebook/dp/B00J2JCZIK.

If you have tried losing weight before, but were unsuccessful, the diet you were using most likely didn't work because you were starving yourself. This leads to you having cravings for food, which leads to a lack of willpower, and you end up gorging yourself. Afterward, you feel guilty about your binge eating and thinking because you blew your diet anyway, you might as well eat yourself into oblivion for that day. Sound familiar? With that diet, you are out of control both emotionally and physically. Stop doing that to yourself!

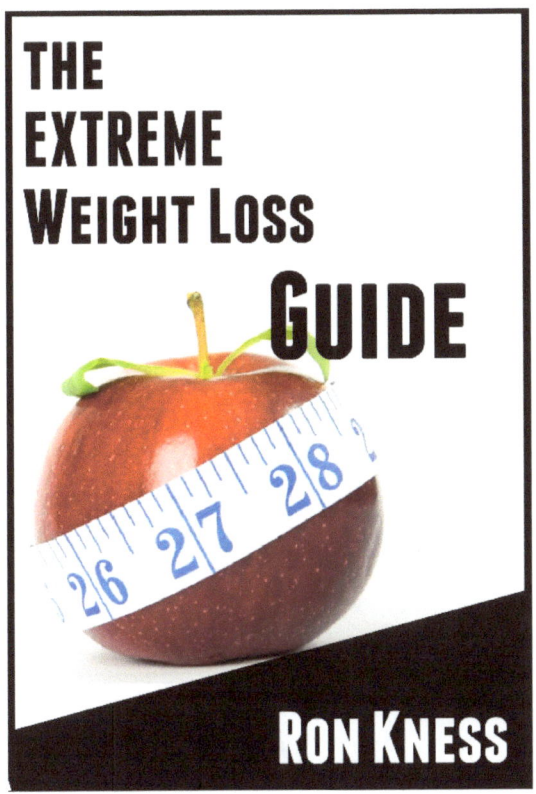

The Extreme Weight Loss Plan
at
http://www.amazon.com/Extreme-Weight-Loss-Plan-Quickly-ebook/dp/B00IRD95FI

Many people struggle with weight loss. They lose weight - the same 20 pounds or more over and over again - only to gain it back over time.
Wouldn't you like to lose that weight forever - and not gain it back.
You can with the information in our plan!

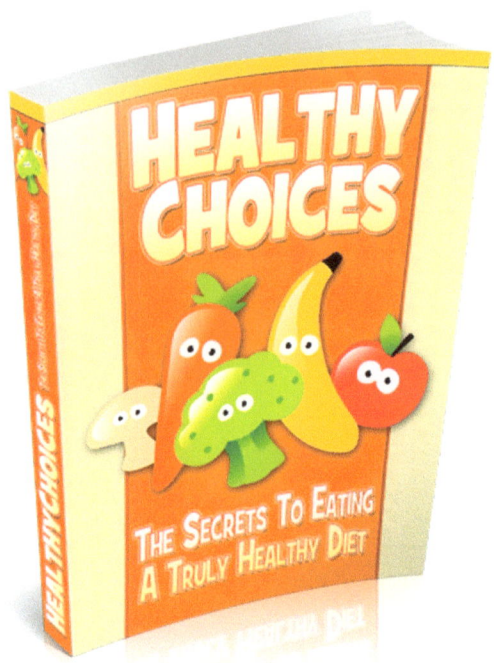

Healthy Choices

at

http://www.jvzoo.com/products/landingpage/9106

Discover The Healthy Eating Secrets You Can Use To Lose Weight & Feel Better Than You Have In Years,

Without Starving Yourself Or Giving Up Your Favorite Foods!

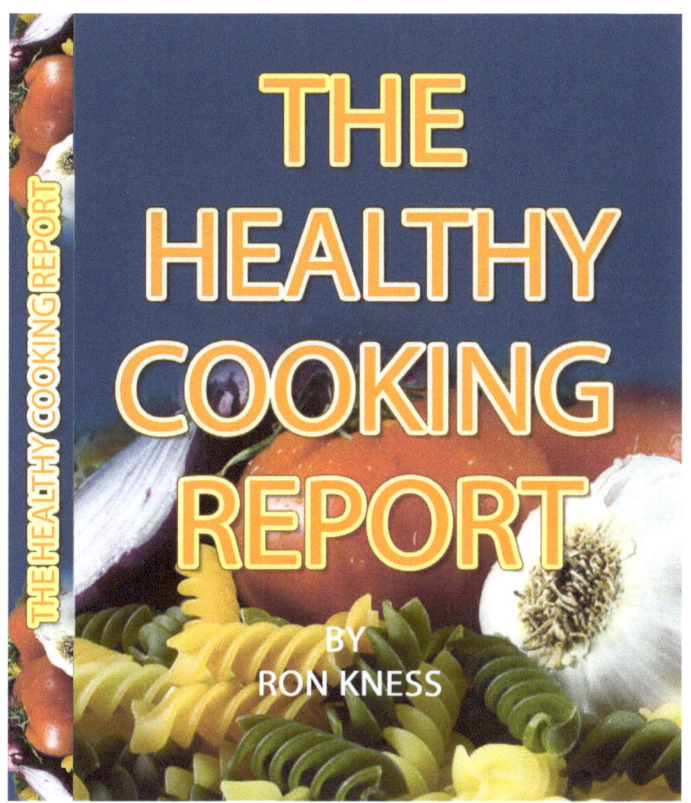

Healthy Cooking

at

http://www.jvzoo.com/products/landingpage/9110

You have decided to change to a healthier lifestyle. Part of making that change involves learning how to cook healthier. In this report,

we show you how to make smart healthy food choices and the best ways to cook them into delicious healthy meals for you and your family.

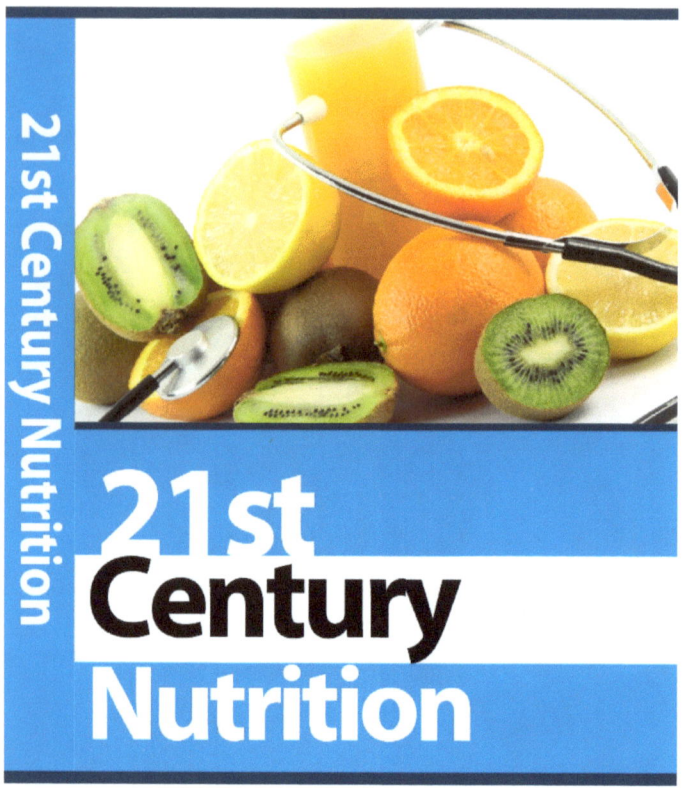

21st Century Nutrition

at

http://www.jvzoo.com/products/landingpage/18526

You have decided to change to a healthier lifestyle. Part of making that change involves learning how to cook healthier.

In this report, we show you how to make smart healthy food choices and the best ways to cook them into delicious healthy meals for you and your family.

For more information on how to lose weight and live the healthy lifestyle, check out our website –

A Healthier You

at

http://healthylifestyle.ronkness.com/home/

About the Author

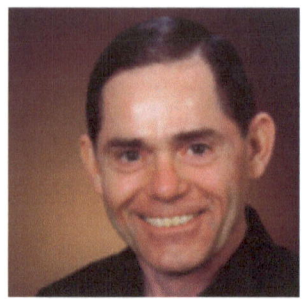

I grew up in Central Minnesota, where my parents own and operated a fishing resort. Once out of high school I tried a couple of semesters of college, only to quit halfway through the Spring term; I decided at that time that college wasn't for me.

Then I decided to follow my father's previous occupation as an auto mechanic. I graduated from a two-year of vocational training course and worked as a mechanic. While in vocational training, I decided to join the National Guard where I eventually ended up working full-time for 32 years.

So how does all of this relate to writing? In one of my leadership schools, the instructor, who was an English teacher at a juvenile detention center, presented writing to me in a whole new way - a way that started to develop my interest in working with words.

Fast forward about 40 years and I now have over 20 books listed on Amazon and CreateSpace. For a complete up-to-date listing, just search for "Ron Kness" (without the quotes of course) in the Kindle Book Store at Amazon.com

www.ingramcontent.com/pod-product-compliance
Lightning Source LLC
Chambersburg PA
CBHW050815290526
45792CB00001B/125